MW00814702

To everyone that helped me walk again.

Plantar Fasciitis Survival Guide
Second Edition

All Rights Reserved.
Copyright © 2014 William Errol Prowse IV

This book may not be reproduced, transmitted, or stored in whole or in part by any means, including graphic, electronic, or mechanical without the express written consent of the publisher except in the case of brief quotations embodied in critical articles and reviews.

ISBN-13: 978-1-50305-024-2

ISBN-10: 1503050246

PRINTED IN THE UNITED STATES OF AMERICA

Medical Disclaimer

The information in this book is not intended or implied to be a substitute for professional medical advice, diagnosis or treatment. All content, including text, graphics, images and information, contained on or available through this book is for general information purposes only. The author makes no representation and assumes no responsibility for the accuracy of information contained on or available through this book, and such information is subject to change without notice. You are encouraged to confirm any information obtained from or through this book with other sources, and review all information regarding any medical condition or treatment with your physician.

NEVER DISREGARD PROFESSIONAL MEDICAL ADVICE OR DELAY SEEKING MEDICAL TREATMENT BECAUSE OF SOMETHING YOU HAVE READ ON OR ACCESSED THROUGH THIS BOOK.

The author does not recommend, endorse or make any representation about the efficacy, appropriateness or suitability of any specific tests, products, procedures, treatments, services, opinions, health care providers or other information that may be contained on or available through this book.

THE AUTHORS IS NEITHER RESPONSIBLE NOR LIABLE FOR ANY ADVICE, COURSE OF TREATMENT, DIAGNOSIS OR ANY OTHER INFORMATION, SERVICES OR PRODUCTS THAT YOU OBTAIN THROUGH THIS BOOK."

Table of Contents

Introduction: You can get rid of your heel pain, but it's going to take some work!

There is no easy way around it: if you have been suffering with the pain of plantar fasciitis, you will do anything to get rid of the pain. This book is made to fix your pain, but you're going to have to work for it. Everything that I show you to fix your pain will have to be done daily until the pain subsides. For some, this will take a couple of weeks. For severe cases, it can take months. This book is laid out in a way that the average person can fix their own plantar fasciitis without knowing any medical jargon. I will lay out the main points, and exactly what to do to fix your own plantar fasciitis at home and without a ton of money.

I had plantar fasciitis for three years straight. My right foot had plantar fasciitis and the left had a partial tear of the plantar fascia. I went to countless doctors and spent tons of money on an endless list of "miracle cures", including stretching devices, ice packs, orthotics, and many others. Nothing worked. Nothing I tried seemed to help, and I was desperate. I am currently a college pre-med student, and felt like the only person that could help me was myself. I talked to doctors about why they couldn't fix me and read a ton of medical literature through my schools databases. I travelled far and wide to "manual soft tissue therapy" practitioners and learned methods that worked. They were hard to find (and expensive), but they were out there. I found what methods really worked on people, and made my very own therapy which I call MSTR (manual soft tissue release).

It took me a long time, but I went from being stuck in bed all day from severe heel pain, to running. I find it hard to understand why expensive doctors couldn't fix me and realized that there are tons of people out there with the same pain as me. This book is made to help you fix your pain. You may be very desperate with your pain, and it is probably ruling your life and thoughts, but plantar fasciitis is not an incurable disease. You can help yourself even if you have had it for a very long time.

Chapter 1: Let's get down to business- Break the habits that are making it worse.

Don't push it

This is simple, but huge. Don't push it, ever. You have a chronic injury that is re-injuring itself on a daily basis. Telling yourself that you are fine and ignoring the pain is setting yourself up for disaster. Even if it means stopping your hobbies and taking time off work, you must do so. If you don't take care of this now, it will get worse and worse until you can't use your foot to walk or even stand. Even if you have had pain for five years straight or more, now is the time to fix it. It is important to accept that if you want this pain to end, you need to make the sacrifices it takes to fix it. Follow my program, and stick with it. You will see results.

Stop taking drugs for inflammation or pain!!

99% of all doctors you meet are going to prescribe you anti- inflammatories to fix your heel pain. Problem with these is that they cause the body not to have any inflammation at all! If you do not have inflammation, you do not have healing. What you want is a strong inflammatory response so that your body can heal your injury. What you don't want is chronic inflammation. Chronic inflammation makes the tissue weaker and doesn't help anything. It's the body's way of "giving up" on an injury. When you take anti-inflammatories, it stops chronic inflammation AND good inflammation.

Another drug you want to stop taking is pain relievers. When you can't feel the pain, you are going to hurt the injured heel even more. This will just make your recovery longer. No matter how much you need to work or keep walking, if you feel too much pain, you HAVE TO REST! If your body tells you something hurts, you need to stop doing it. It's as simple as that.

One way of stopping the chronic inflammation cycle is to have a good diet. This includes stopping consumption of meats and sugars. Two great supplements for chronic inflammation will be mentioned in great detail later are systemic enzymes and fish oil. Check out my diet chapter to know how to use these.

Tip toeing is not helping

It may feel as if it is reducing pain in the heel, but this will cause much more pain in the long run! Tip toeing causes the plantar fascia to have more tension and could cause more tearing. It also causes a limp, and that alone makes the hips/knees and rest of the body to be negatively affected.

How to fix this:

Stop doing it! This is a VERY hard habit to break if you have been doing it for months, but you can overcome it. You may be wondering, "that's crazy! If I don't tip toe I will scream in pain because it will feel like a nail is going through my heel!". And that is why you will learn to use athletic tape. Jump to the chapter on taping if you are in severe pain and can't stand to tip toe. If not, stop tip toeing now!

Don't stop moving

I understand the pain can be HUGE, but that is no excuse to stop moving! When you stop moving, wastes accumulate around the injury and cause lots of negative effects to the body's healing ability. When you move, even a little bit, your whole body pumps blood and nutrients into the injury and pumps out the wastes. If you move, you speed up healing immensely.

How to fix this:

Active Rest

One thing you can't do is sit around waiting for your plantar fasciitis to heal. You need to find what you can do that doesn't hurt your plantar fasciitis. Some of my personal top picks are swimming, bicycling, and working out the upper body/core. Staying active during recovery is a great way to stay sane and increase blood flow to the plantar fascia. If you know something hurts, don't do it. This maybe a very simple concept, but as time goes by you may feel like you're not getting better, and will try things out of desperation from all the frustration. Just don't. You get one chance to heal properly, so don't test things that you know will hurt. If you know you screwed up and hurt it more, bust out the ice.

Keep the foot moving

 If you cannot get out of bed because of the pain, move your foot in every way possible. Point your toes and then bring them back up (flexing toes toward the shin). Do this AS MUCH AS YOU CAN. This causes the veins in the legs to literally "pump" blood to the injury. This will make it heal faster. Move the foot in every direction that's COMFORTABLE TO YOU. Some movements will not feel that great, so don't push those, but for any movement that doesn't hurt should be done daily. If you can't walk twenty minutes, walk ten. DO NOT GIVE UP! Keep everything moving!

Do not depend on doctors to always fix your pain

There are no miracle cures for every case of plantar fasciitis. No matter how great of a doctor you have, most will have difficulty treating a bad case of plantar fasciitis. You are your own best therapist when it comes to treating plantar fasciitis.

Tip: Read into every treatment the doctor suggests before getting it done. Surgeries for plantar fasciitis have horrible outcomes from most of the information I have read. Cortisone shots give temporary relief but weakens the plantar fascia over time. My opinion is to go to a trained soft tissue therapist. The next best hope is a doctor who specializes in ESWT. This is hard to come by in the USA but in Canada it is cheap and easily found (I went there twice and had some degree of "help" from it, but not lasting relief, what worked best is what I will show you soon.)

Try to stay positive

This one is extremely difficult. If you told me to stay positive when I couldn't walk for 5 months, I would have started to laugh at you, then cry. Plantar fasciitis is a beast, and most people and doctors you talk to will never understand your pain, and will look at you like you are crazy. Ignore these people and give it everything you've got to fix your feet.

Chapter 2: Diet

If you eat a lot of sugar/fast food/trans fats (hydrogenated oils)/excessive salt, your heel pain will not heal nearly as fast. Because everyone's bodies are different, I will just list basics such as what to eat. If it's not on the list, it's better to avoid it completely. After the food list, I will show you some supplements that can give your body's healing powers a boost.

What you can eat:

o **All fruits and vegetables.** Avoid dried fruit/fruit juices. Also avoid the "night shade" plants. These promote chronic inflammation and include tomatoes, white potatoes, and bell peppers.

o **All nuts and seeds.** These are best raw. Avoid the roasted/salted nuts and seeds. Try to add ground flaxseed to your diet. This seed has tons of great nutrients that help fight chronic inflammation. Try to include as many nut and seed sprouts as possible.

o **Whole grains only**. No refined flours like white wheat flour. Some good examples are: quinoa, oatmeal, millet, amaranth, brown rice, barley, buckwheat, spelt, rye, whole grain wheat. (The less grains the better, even whole grains. I know how hard this is for some people so I am leaving it on the list. But keep in mind that the most ideal choice is to not consume grains at all).

- **All spices and herbs**

- **Some meats.** Chicken, turkey, and venison are ok in moderation. It's also best to avoid these as well if you can.

- **All seafood**. Especially Wild Alaskan Salmon.

Note: Avoid sugar; instead use stevia, black strap molasses, honey, and maple syrup. I recommend only stevia. All the other sweeteners must be used in extreme moderation. It's best to avoid them entirely if possible.

I understand that when you change someone's diet, it's almost as radical as changing their religion. Most people look at this diet plan and say "no way can I do that!". It's up to you if you want your heel to heal faster, and following this diet can do wonders. So try your best to follow the guidelines above.

If you want a more "complete" diet for pain, check out my newest book called "The Chronic Pain and Systemic Inflammation Diet" available now on amazon.com.

The Food List

These are the most ideal foods to eat when you have plantar fasciitis.

Vegetables:

- Arugula
- Asparagus
- Avocado
- Beets
- Broccoli
- Capers
- Cauliflower
- Crookneck squash
- Cucumbers
- Fennel bulb
- Horseradish
- Leek
- Lettuce (All Kinds)
- Kale
- Mushrooms
- Mustard greens
- Onions
- Sweet Potatoes or Yams
- Spinach
- Swiss chard
- Watercress
- Yams
- Celery

Sprouts

- Alfalfa
- Broccoli
- Buckwheat
- Mung Bean
- Red clover
- Fenugreek
- Mustard seed
- Wheat Grass
- Sunflower

Berries

- Bilberry
- Blackberry
- Boysenberry
- Cranberry
- Hawthorne berry
- Juniper berry
- Loganberry
- Mulberry
- Raspberry
- Red currant
- Strawberry

Fruits

- Apricot
- Cherries
- Coconut
- Figs
- Guava
- Honeydew melon
- Kiwi
- Lemon
- Lime
- Mandarin orange
- Nectarine
- Olives
- Papaya
- Passion fruit
- Peach
- Pear
- Persimmon
- Pineapple
- Plum
- Pomegranate (Raw only, not the juice they sell in stores!)
- Star fruit
- Tangerine
- Rhubarb

Herbs / Spices

- Allspice
- Anise
- Basil
- Bay leaf
- Cayenne
- Chamomile
- Chives
- Cilantro
- Cinnamon
- Cloves
- Cumin
- Dill
- Elephant garlic
- Fenugreek
- Ginger
- Hawthorne leaf
- Marigold flowers
- Marjoram
- Mustard (seed, leaf)
- Noni
- Nutmeg
- Oregano
- Paprika
- Peppermint
- Rosemary
- Sage
- Spearmint
- Tarragon
- Thyme
- Turmeric
- Vanilla bean
- Yucca

Miscellaneous

- Nutritional Yeast Flakes
- Sauerkraut (Only Raw. Most on the market are not)
- Spirulina
- Pickled Vegetables
- Apple Cider Vinegar
- Fresh/Raw Wheat Grass Juice

Natural Sweeteners

- Stevia

Nuts and Seeds

- Walnuts
- Almonds
- Sunflower seeds
- Flaxseed
- Pumpkin seeds
- Brazil nuts

- Anise seed
- Pine nuts
- Cashews
- Fennel seed
- Caraway seed
- Sesame seeds

Protein Sources

- Almonds
- Wild Alaskan Salmon
- Mushrooms
- Sprouts
- Pumpkin Seeds
- Sprouts

Great Fatty Acid Oils (Must be Extra Virgin/Cold Pressed)

- Avocado Oil
- Apricot Kernel Oil

- Almond Oil
- Flaxseed Oil
- Olive Oil
- Hazelnut Oil
- Walnut Oil

Medicinal Herbs

- Angelica
- Aloe
- Ashwagandha
- Black Cohosh
- Circumin
- Devils Claw
- Fever Few
- Turmeric (1st Favorite)
- Boswellia (2nd Favorite)
- White Poplar
- White Willow Bark (3rd Favorite)
- Winter Green
- Wormwood

Supplements

These are going to be listed in order from most important to least important. When you take them all at the same time, they work together synergistically to boost your results. Some are expensive, but well worth the money.

Fish oil: I suggest 1000-3000 mg a day. I have heard of people taking up to 9,000 mg a day for the anti-inflammatory affect to kick in. Fish oil is famous for its anti-inflammatory properties, and can help you greatly in the long run.

Systemic enzymes: These are an amazing supplement, and they give the body the ability to break free of the previously talked about "chronic inflammation". These go through your blood and break down scar tissue and absorb and destroy chemicals that are causing the chronic inflammation. There are many on the market, but Wobenzyme® has the best reviews of them all and is what I use on a daily basis. These pills are expensive, but well worth the money. It's best to start with 3 pills, 3 times a day, slowly increasing your dose to 7 pills, 3 times a day. When your pain has decreased at least 20-30 percent, you can decrease your dose back down to 3 pills, 3 times a day. I have heard of people taking 12 pills, 3 times a day, with great results. The number one most important rule for taking these is to take them on a completely EMPTY stomach and do not eat until an hour has passed after taking them.

MSM: This one is cheap, and very effective for pain relief. It works by pushing nutrients through the many membranes in your body, and allows for faster healing because of this mechanism. It also has a huge list of other benefits, so many in fact, that people have written books on just this supplement alone. I suggest 1000 mg a day, but you can take as much as 5000mg if you are in severe pain.

Vitamin D3: Another cheap vitamin with tons of benefits. Over 90 percent of Americans are deficient in this vitamin alone, and if you do not have enough of it, it can be the number one cause of your heel spur if you have one. Start off with 5000 I.U.s daily and try to take it for as long as you can. This vitamin is so cheap that there is no reason anyone shouldn't take it.

Magnesium Citrate/Calcium Citrate: Only cheap if you buy from Costco/Amazon.com. This supplement helps with bone growth and repair, but it also has neurological benefits (having to do with the nerves). Muscles depend on calcium to contract, and they also depend on magnesium to relax. If you are at all deficient in these vitamins, beating plantar fasciitis will be much harder. I suggest 1000 mg daily of the calcium citrate, and 400 mg of the magnesium citrate.

Multivitamin: The cheapest way to get a ton of vitamins. There is a ton on the market, but I suggest Opti-Men from Optimum Nutrition®. They have great reviews and I love them.

Vitamin E: Supports a healthy inflammatory response and is needed by tons of chemical reactions in the body. Take the recommended dosage mentioned on the bottle.

Water

Increase your water intake and you will see major benefits! When the plantar fascia is constantly inflamed, it is making a lot of waste products. The fastest way to expel these from the body is to drink a lot of water. It also makes your connective tissue (fascia) a lot more supple and able to be stretched and healed.

There are many recommendations on how much water to drink. I recommend everyone to take a water bottle with them and drink as much as they feel comfortable drinking. This seems like a simple and basic step, but it can help a lot.

Chapter 3: A rough overview of what's to come

The main treatment method in my program is a combination of stretching and something called manual soft tissue release (MSTR). MSTR is a name I give to a method created by combining techniques from all the popular soft tissue manipulation therapies. Each of these methods are used to release soft tissue in some way. My method combines them in the most effective way to beat plantar fasciitis.

Why release soft tissue? What is soft tissue?

Soft tissue belongs to anything that isn't bone/cartilage and usually refers to muscles, tendons, ligaments, and fascia (this connects everything together). When an injury happens in the body, these structures tighten up, which makes it difficult to move the injured area of the body. All the soft tissue around the injury stays tight, often even after the injury has healed. When everything is tight, and we move the injured/healed area, it will re-injure itself. This causes a horrible downward spiral and the injury keeps hurting itself over and over.

These tight areas also slow down nutrient flow, reducing the healing rate. If this cycle continues for a long enough time, your body starts chronic inflammatory responses instead of healing responses. When this happens, the body literally gives up on "healing" and starts to break the area down, making it even weaker. Eventually, it may seem that the pain is impossible to cure, and that you will be in a never-ending cycle of pain and injury. There is a way to break free from this.

22

MSTR addresses all of these issues. First, it releases the tight muscles so that the injured area gets a chance to heal. It forces nutrients into the injury. It also frees the restrictions that feed the area with nutrients (compressed nerves/lymphatic flow/blood flow). Some MSTR methods also cause a forced inflammatory response which leads to immediate healing in the area, breaking the chronic inflammation cycle. It causes cell growth in the area and forces the body to lay down new collagen fibers in the injury to strength it. This is what you need to focus on:

- The muscles/tendons that compose the calf muscle are tight

- The muscles/tendons/ligaments going from the heel to the toes are tight

- The muscles/tendons of the hamstrings are tight

- MSTR is needed for the injured area to break free of the chronic inflammation cycle

What's the fastest way to fix this problem?

1. Support the plantar fascia with athletic tape. I had to do this every day for 8 months just to be able to walk. Taping takes some of the stress off the plantar fascia so it can have a better chance at healing. This helps enable you to keep on moving without nearly as much limping/pain. It is really hard to become proficient at taping early on, so keep trying the taping methods until you have some relief. It can take a while to learn a method that works for you. Most people will always be able to find relief with taping; it's just very hard to tape plantar fasciitis properly. Skip ahead to the chapter on taping to find out how this is done.

2. Support the plantar fascia with an orthotic. I recommend the brand called "Super Feet". Everyone's feet are different, and if you want to find one that works for your feet, you usually have to try a lot of them. Custom orthotics are a good option if you can afford them.

3. Deactivate all trigger points with MSTR. This is done through a form of massage where you feel your foot, calf, and hamstring for tender areas, and apply rubbing pressure till they are not as tender. These "trigger points" are responsible for most of the pain you experience.

4. Free restrictions in the connective tissue with MSTR. This is done by scraping the muscles with different tools that you will make with things around your house.

5. Special stretches made specifically for treating plantar fasciitis. These need to be done every day, but ONLY after you have fixed the trigger points and restrictions in the connective tissue.

6. Cause a localized inflammatory response to break the chronic inflammation cycle that your body has adopted in response to having plantar fasciitis for an extended amount of time. This also gives the body the ability to lay down new fibers and restructure the weakened areas of the injury. This step is usually done with focused rubbing with a tool. These will be outlined in the "bonus MSTR methods" section.

Things to keep in mind:

- Stretching a muscle that has trigger points or severely tight fascia (the connective tissue that joins all the muscle fibers together) will cause more damage! You must release these trigger points first and stretch the muscle second to make the changes permanent. This is often a leading cause for why traditional physical therapy fails for chronic cases of plantar fasciitis.

- If a stretch or method hurts more than 6 out of 10 on the pain scale, you need to stop! Try again but much slower and/or with less pressure.

- A lot of stretches prescribed by physical therapists can do more harm than good. They put the plantar fascia under extreme stress and don't focus on the soft tissue around the injury (the trigger points and tight fascia) that is the actual cause of the plantar fasciitis not being able to heal. Once you get rid of the perpetuating factors, the body can heal the plantar fascia pretty quickly.

- When you feel a healthy muscle without trigger points, it has a consistent texture; it is soft and supple and easy to grab and massage. In a muscle with trigger points and tight fascia, it will have a grainy texture and will be harder than a healthy muscle. It will also have little pea sized lumps and taut bands running throughout the length of the muscle. Our goal is to get rid of these.

- You won't get better unless you work for it. There are no magical cures for plantar fasciitis. Positive thinking and hope are not going to fix your pain. You need to fix the problems causing your plantar fasciitis and carry on with your life.

Chapter 4: MSTR- The daily step by step methods to fix your heel pain!

Here is a brief summary of the daily methods that you need to complete at least once a day. I highly recommend doing only steps 1 and 2 for the first 2-3 weeks:

1. Find tender trigger points and massage them out.

2. Release the connective tissue (fascia) by scraping it with a tool you will find around the house (much more on this later).

3. After doing step 1 and 2 for some time (2-3 weeks), the tissues will feel different in the foot and lower leg. They are finally ready to be stretched. You will have a few stretches to do every day which are described in the following chapters.

4. Bonus MSTR methods that are done once or twice a week to break free of the chronic inflammation cycle.

5. After doing the program for about 6 weeks, you will know exactly which methods/stretches that help the most. Continue these until you are back to normal.

How long until I see results from MSTR?

Keep in mind that everyone's plantar fasciitis is very different. If you are overweight and have had it for a long time, it's going to be extremely hard to get rid of. Some people can have fantastic recoveries from MSTR shortly after starting. I suggest that after 2-3 weeks of doing trigger point therapy/scraping, you will notice some difference no matter how bad your case is. Once you move on to the rest of the methods, you will notice that your recovery is predictable, and this is where I want you to be. I want you to know that it is getting better and stronger day by day, and that there is a light at the end of the tunnel.

How fast should I progress through the methods of MSTR?

For the first 2-3 weeks, you should only do trigger point work and scraping (steps one and two). You should "ease" into these treatments. Go very carefully with these treatments at first until your body is used to them. It is more ideal to do multiple "light pressure" trigger point/ scraping treatment sessions every day, than to have one "hard pressure" session once a day.

After the trigger points are released and the fascia is unrestricted, you will have a new understanding of what is causing your pain and how you can fix it yourself. When you feel comfortable with first two steps, you are ready to move on. Your muscles and ligaments will feel different and your pain should be lower. This is when you know you are ready to stretch.

Some of you may try one of the methods and find that you get instant relief. That's great! I found myself getting the most relief from scraping and using a wooden roller. Some of you will have better relief from doing just trigger point massages with a lacrosse ball. If you feel that one of the methods is helping you more than the other ones, stick to it and forget my guidelines and do what feels good! Just be sure to give all the methods a solid chance and be sure to follow my guidelines in the step by step order I outlined first and foremost.

Step One: Find Trigger Points and Massage Them Out

Three tools are needed:

- o Hands/Knee/Knuckles

- o Wooden Roller

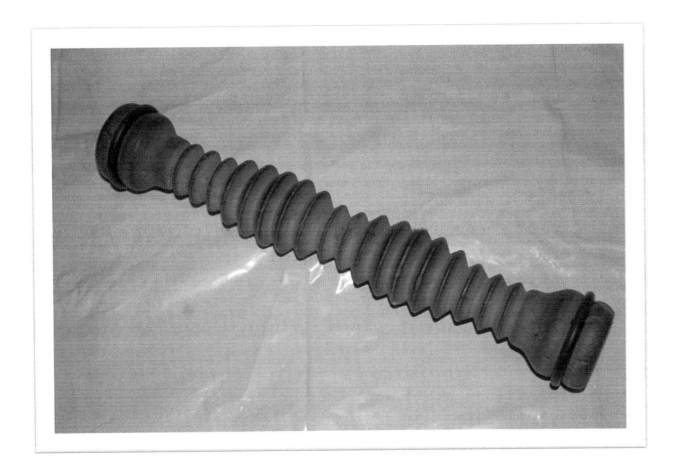

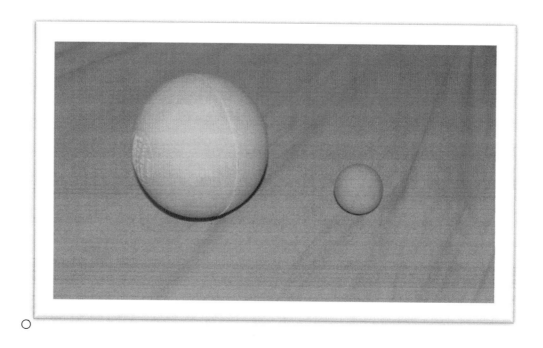

o Lacrosse ball/ Computer mouse ball (these are hard to find but the best. If you cannot find a computer mouse ball, get a "super bouncy" rubber ball that is often sold in candy machines in grocery stores).

Some trigger point guidelines:

You will use these tools to "deactivate" the trigger points in your calves and foot. Trigger points are tender spots of tissue in the muscle that are made in response to any and all injuries in the body. Their purpose is to cause pain when you move your foot/ankle. This is to force you to rest so that your body can fix the damage in the heel. These trigger points are great for fixing injures and forcing someone to rest, but if you have chronic plantar fasciitis (anything over six weeks) the trigger points are causing you more harm than good.

The best way to find these trigger points is to feel around the foot and calf for tender spots that hurt to rub. Sometimes it will have a "good pain" like when you get knots massaged out of your back. The key to releasing trigger points is to not apply too much pressure. It's best not to go more than 6 out of 10 on the pain scale, where 0 is no pain, and 10 is the most pain.

Using the tools will allow you to use more pressure on a trigger point than you can with just your hands.

The pictures in the following pages will show guidelines to where common trigger points will be (they will be red dots in the pictures). Your job is to find them and rub them out until they are not as "tender".

Some people will have to hit all the trigger points; some will only have a couple. Sometimes you will not only find a tender spot, but you might find a small nodule or lump or tight band in the muscle as well. This is good! You need to slowly massage this out until it is not as tender as when you started. Rubbing them back and forth is the best way to do this. Rub them nice and slow. If you apply too much pressure to these little trigger points, you will have more pain / problems. If you massage them nice and softly and have a medium amount of pain while doing so, you will have less pain / problems with your plantar fasciitis. If you do not feel a tender spot, try pushing harder / deeper into the tissues. Sometimes they like to hide pretty deep inside a muscle.

One extra thing to know about trigger points is that they cause "referred pain patterns". This means that when you have active trigger points in your calves your body will automatically send pain signals to your heel, even if the plantar fascia is already healed. This is why I suggest doing these first to see what kind of results you get. For some, these trigger point methods will practically "fix" you. For most, they need to be done consistently until your heel pain is gone.

After a few sessions of trigger point therapy, you may feel like your tender spots have become less sensitive and that you might be fine without any more trigger point work. This is so wrong. Keep feeling around the muscles and search for new trigger points. Sometimes after doing the superficial (surface) layer of muscles, you will later find a whole new set of trigger points deeper in the muscle. These ones will usually require more applied pressure to release, so if you are not seeing results, try pushing a bit harder. Just keep with it daily and do not give up!

You can do these trigger point release methods any time throughout the day. If you are in a lot of pain, doing them 6 times a day is fine (6 light sessions is better than 1 intense session a day). If the area becomes extremely sore or feels more tender, let the area rest and come back to it in a day or two. Your body will adapt to the therapy quickly, and it is not unusual for you to be able to double the amount of therapy sessions and pressure that you use on the trigger points in as little as 2-3 weeks. It is important to slowly ease into the treatments and to build up to more sessions / more applied pressure while massaging. Listen to your body.

If you want to see how these methods are done, check out my video tutorial on how to release these trigger points. Go to an internet browser and type this into your address bar:

http://www.pfsurvivalguide.com/trigger-point-tutorial

Time to get started! The next page will have your first set of common trigger points.

Trigger point set number one:

Common Calf Trigger points:

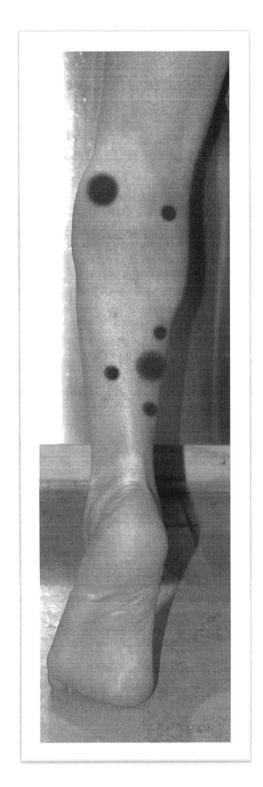

Methods to massage Set One:

Use the opposite legs knee to push into your calf as shown in the picture below. This should be one of your main methods of massaging the calf muscle trigger points. I like to search over the entire calf muscle for trigger points with this method because it is easy to feel around with your knee for tender spots (trigger points).

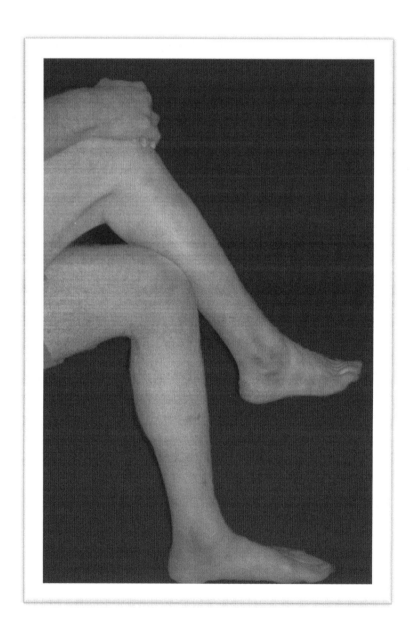

Another method is to press your knuckles straight into the calf muscle. This is a great method for rubbing out a trigger point ONLY if you know where they are. I like using the previous "knee massage" method to find them, and I love using this one to rub them out. This method is great for getting rid of huge trigger points if you find them.

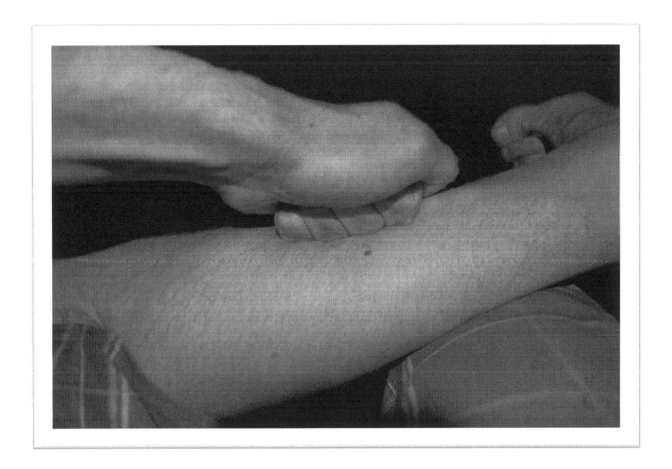

The last method is to use your fingers to press the trigger points. This method does not apply nearly as much pressure as the last two methods, but you can feel the tissues extremely well with your fingers and thumbs. This is when you can feel tiny nodules in the muscle and rub directly on them. I like to cross my legs so I can reach the muscles easier with my hands.

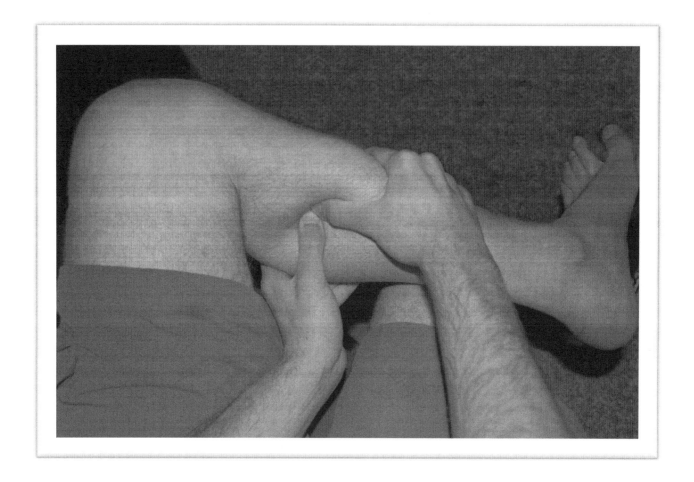

Trigger point set number two:

Common foot trigger points

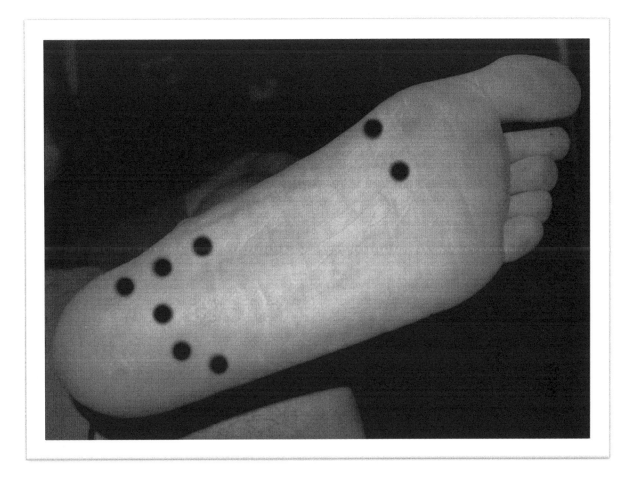

This massage ball will be your new best friend for trigger point massage! These things are great for rubbing out the tender spots you will find all over the bottom of your foot (trigger point set #2). Once you feel comfortable massaging the tender spots on the bottom of the foot with the lacrosse ball, use a smaller ball, such as a "super bouncy" rubber ball (as shown below). I prefer lacrosse balls because they keep their "grip" and do not wear out easily.

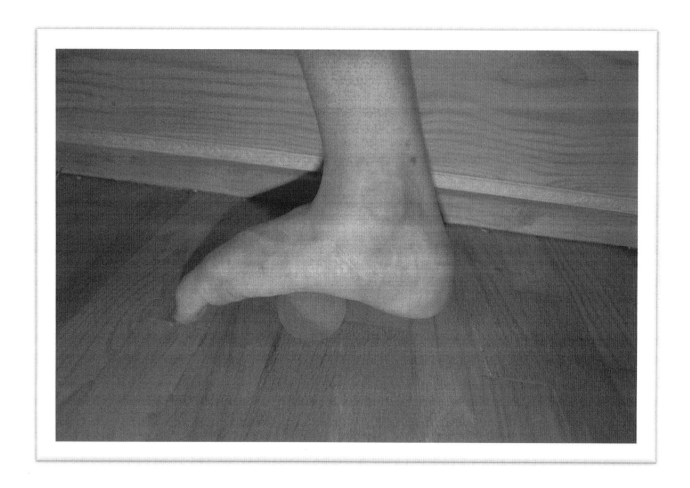

Massage therapy foot rollers are worth every penny and will help you a ton. If you are on a budget, this is the most important tool. I have a cheap and quality foot roller posted on my website (www.pfsurvivalguide.com) under the "Helpful Tools" section.

Part One

First, start with a few light passes with the foot roller to warm up the tissues that are getting massaged. Just go back and forth over the whole bottom of your foot. After a short while, it will not hurt nearly as much. For some, this can take a long time. If my foot is in a lot of pain, I will sit at my computer rolling my foot over it lightly to warm it up. Sometimes it only takes me a minute to warm it up; other times, it takes much longer. When the foot feels less general pain, you are ready to go to the next step.

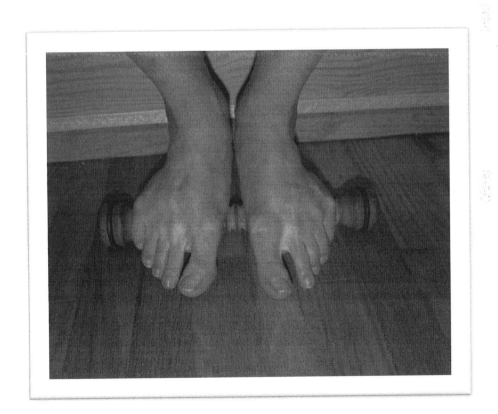

Part Two

Now we will do some serious work with the foot roller. First we need to hit every part of the foot. We will do this in three different ways. First, we will do the very bottom of the foot by flexing the toes to the sky. Go back and forth over the whole foot until you find a tender spot and massage it out the best that you can. You may even feel a lump right in front of the heel (the back portion of the arch). This lump usually causes people a lot of pain, and needs to be rubbed out as much as possible. It may feel incredibly painful to do this at first, but the relief it brings is incredible! These massages are typically most helpful after a long period of sitting or just before getting out of bed in the morning. It may take you a while to do this exercise with your toes pointed up. Make this your goal and try to work toward it as quickly as you can. Be soft and gentle for the first few sessions, your body needs time to adapt to this treatment.

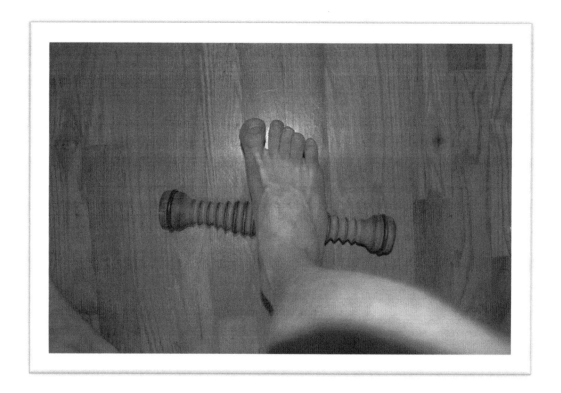

Part Three

Next, we want to get the outside edge of the foot. Most of this area is bone, but the soft portions are usually filled with trigger points. Try to rub the outside edge of the heel itself. You may even feel a lump around or on the heel. Try to rub this out nice and slowly with moderate pressure. It will eventually feel less tender; this is when you can increase pressure.

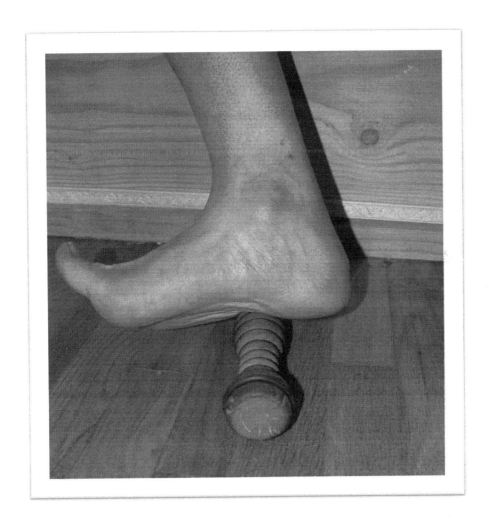

Part Four

The last pass you need to do is the inner edge of the foot. This will probably be very tender for most and is hard to do during your fist attempt. Go nice and easy at first and increase the pressure if it is comfortable to do so.

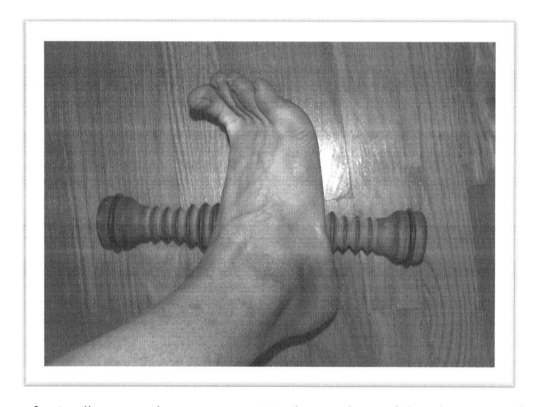

These foot roller exercises are great to do anytime of the day, and I feel were a huge reason that my plantar fasciitis has not come back. They will be painful to do at first, but ease into it and stick with it for best results.

The next step of MSTR: releasing fascia through scraping tools

This one a bit tricky, but once you master this technique; it will set you up for a LOT of relief from your plantar fasciitis. This method also makes the results you see from your trigger point releasing more "permanent" and gives the trigger points less reason to come back.

Why release the fascia?

The trigger points we released earlier are bundles of muscle fibers that are held tight in a chronically contracted state. Around these muscle fibers, there is connective tissue (fascia) that structurally holds the muscle fibers together. When the trigger points are locked in place for a long time, the fascia tightens around the trigger points until the fascia is tight as well. The fascia needs to be released if you want your trigger point therapy results to stay. Once you release the trigger points, it is MUCH easier to release the fascia. The way we do this is by scraping the tissues with a plastic edge. What you want is something that can apply very direct pressure to a tissue, but not damage the skin.

Check out my video tutorial for scraping to get a better idea of what to do. Go online and type this address into your browser:
http://www.pfsurvivalguide.com/scraping-tutorial

Scraping guidelines:

The muscles need to be relaxed in order to release the fascia around them. This is done by contracting the opposite side of the body part you are working with. When you release the calf muscle fascia, you need to make sure your shin muscle is contracted. To do this, bring the top of your foot as high up as you can toward the shin. This will stretch the calf muscle and make it easier to scrape. When you release the bottom of the foot's fascia, you need to pull your toes back as far as you can with one hand, then scrape the bottom of the foot with the other hand.

USE LUBRICATION: any lotion will work usually. Put it all over the area being treated. DO NOT SCRAPE WITHOUT!

The pictures will show "start" and "end" positions for where to use the tools. Use equal pressure over the whole area, and scrape the whole thing. The end goal is to do a few passes with moderate pressure. Do a few light pressure passes first and slowly build up to moderate pressure. After a few sessions of scraping, you can build up to more extreme amounts of pressure. Try to go a little harder each time. This does not mean hurt yourself! Just do what is comfortable, but be a bit aggressive with the pressure. Even if it feels really good to scrape, do not scrape more than 10-20 times. The best rule of thumb is to stop when the area is less tender.

Do these every day after one of your trigger point therapy sessions, but not as often as the trigger point therapies. Even if you are doing 6 sessions of trigger point therapy, do only 1 session of scraping. Once your body adapts to this therapy, you will be able to increase the amount of sessions / amount of pressure applied. If anything feels more tender or sore, take a day or two of rest, and ease back into it.

You will probably hear noises when you scrape the muscles, this is good! It means that you are finding adhesions in the tissue and are releasing them.

The texture that you will look for in the tissues is a "grainy" texture. If you were to scrape over a healthy muscle instead, it will feel nice and smooth. When you scrape a muscle that has tight fascia (this is bad and is caused from your Plantar Fasciitis), it will feel rough and grainy from all the adhesions. These are where you want to focus your pressure. Try to rub out the grains by passing the tools more over these areas.

Tools for scraping:

I love using a spatula, but plastic cutting boards work as well. The most important thing you need in your scraping tool is something with a plastic edge, and it shouldn't be able to cut the skin. Try to find something a few millimeters thick. The edge of a spatula, the part you cook with, is great for scraping. Other objects, such as plastic cutting boards work extremely well, and have a dull / rounded plastic edge. The dull / rounded edge works really well when first starting out. Use some common sense and creativity and you should be able to find something around the house.

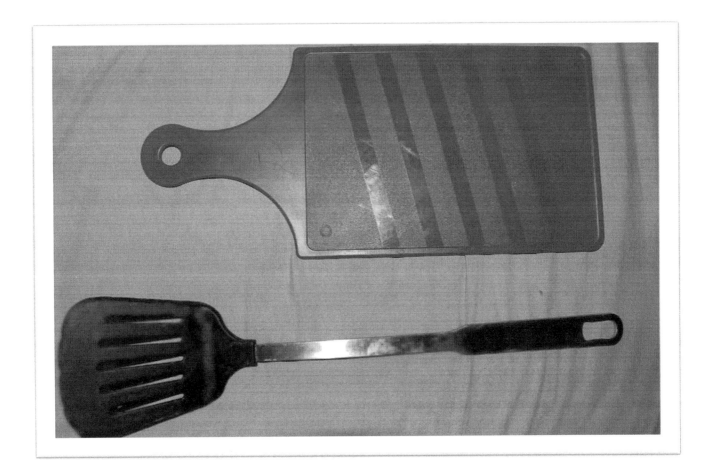

This is the edge that we are looking for: a dull, round plastic edge.

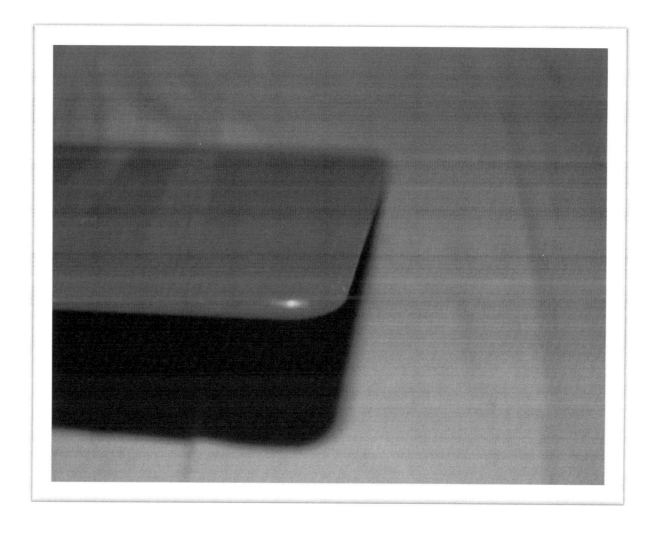

First area to start scraping:

Use one of the tools above to scrape from the bottom of the Achilles tendon, and up to where the calf muscle bulges out (half way up the lower leg). Try to stretch the calf muscle by lifting the foot toward the knee cap, and then scrape the Achilles tendon area. As is the same with the roller, you need to get all areas of this area being treated. Try to scrape the outside edge of the Achilles tendon, the inside edge, and the middle. This area can make a lot of noise. This may be scary and somewhat painful at first, but it is a huge "problem causer" when it comes to heel pain. Start with very light pressure, and slowly build up. I suggest using a very dull / rounded plastic edged tool for this one.

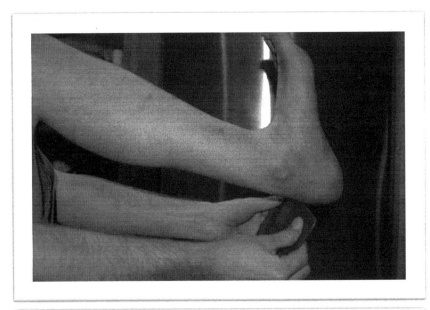

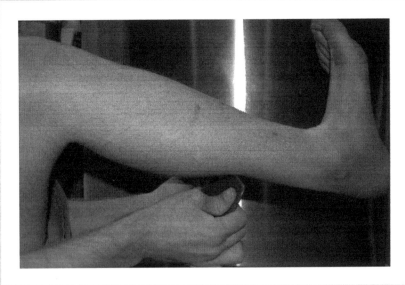

The second area to scrape:

Next we will scrape the bottom of the foot. When you do this area, it is important to get EVERY PART scraped. Some good places to scrape are the arch of the foot, right behind the big toe joint, and right in front of the heel. With this you will need to scrape every angle of the foot, but try to always start at the toes, and scrape all the way back towards the heel. Experiment and try to find tender / tight spots. Not all spots are the same, and you have to "search and destroy" the tender spots/tight fascia. When working on the bottom of the foot, I suggest using a spatula, or a tool with a sharper edge.

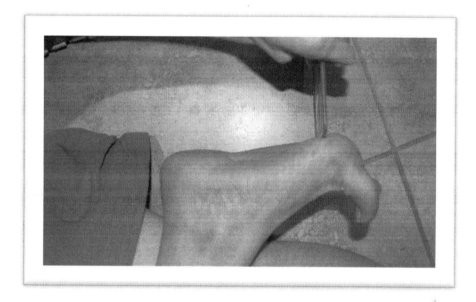

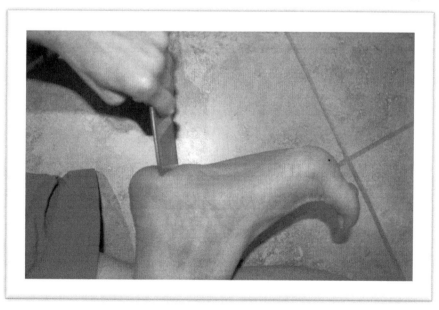

The third area to scrape:

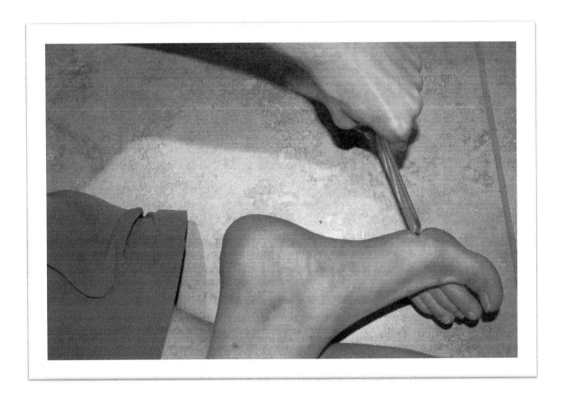

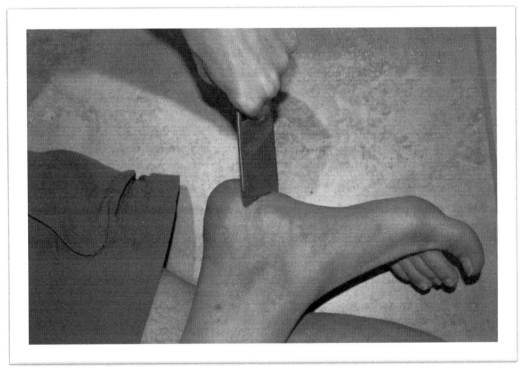

The fourth area to scrape:

Most of this area is bone, but there is a soft section right in front of the heel. This area may be small, but it has a lot of tight fascia. After I got the hang of releasing this area, I had tons of pain relief. I was overlooking this area for weeks. Go over this area a few times to see if there is any tight fascia there.

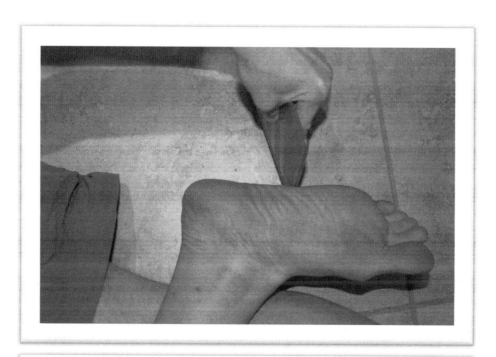

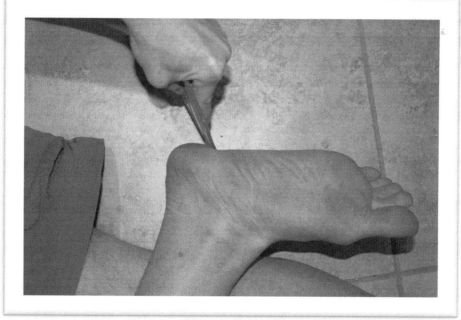

Time for stretching!

Remember: never stretch unless you have taken care of those cumbersome trigger points! Don't forget that you need to do just the trigger point / scraping methods for about 2-3 weeks before you start most of these stretches. Here are the stretching guidelines:

○ Never stretch a cold muscle! You HAVE to warm up those muscles before you stretch. If you don't, you can wind up hurting yourself even more. This can be very difficult if you have plantar fasciitis, because you obviously can't run. Some nice options instead are to bicycle or swim. I like to make sure I am at least out of breath from bicycling, and then I know I'm ready to go.

○ These stretches are made so that you must follow every step. If you don't, you can stress joints and cause further damage. It's much more effective if you stretch the fascia as opposed to muscle. In order to do this, you need to stretch a whole group of muscles in what's called a "kinetic chain". For plantar fasciitis, you need to stretch the bottom of the foot, the calf, the hamstring, and the lower back all at once! So again, make sure you follow all the instructions for each stretch so that you stretch the fascia and not the muscles.

○ If something hurts, STOP! These stretches are very focused and have a VERY specific purpose. If something feels more painful than a "pull", you need to stop. Always ease into each stretch nice and very slowly. Even if you have been doing the stretches for weeks, you need to still warm up and go into them slowly to avoid causing damage.

A lot of these stretches require contraction (flexing) of a muscle group. This is because when you contract one muscle, another muscle has to relax in order for it to do so. When you have the muscle fibers relaxed, they are not being pulled / stretched, so instead, it will stretch the connective tissue around the muscle. This is the fascia that keeps getting mentioned, and is the reason we are stretching.

Again, do not attempt these stretches until a few weeks after you have been doing the trigger point therapy, with one exception. Stretch number one is the only one that I want you to start today, right now, and do it every day until your pain subsides. Make sure to do this one before getting out of bed every morning. It does not stress the muscles/joints as much as other stretches and it is more of a "warm up movement" than an actual "stretch".

Check out my video demonstration for these stretches. Go online and type this address into your browser:
http://www.pfsurvivalguide.com/plantar-fasciitis-stretches

Stretch One

Part One

Isolate the big toe, and pull it back. Hold for 30 seconds.

This stretch and the next two toe stretches do not require you to be warmed up. They are the only stretches that can be done at any time of the day.

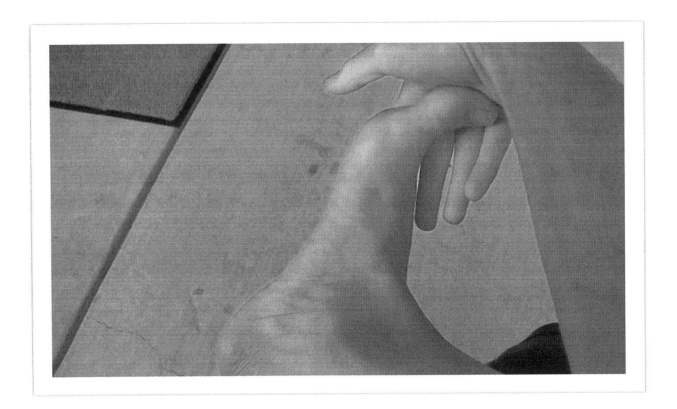

Part Two

Grab all the toes and pull them back. Try to go as far back as you can. For some of you, the big toe will be harder to pull back, and for others, the other toes will be harder to pull back. This is how you grab them for the stretch:

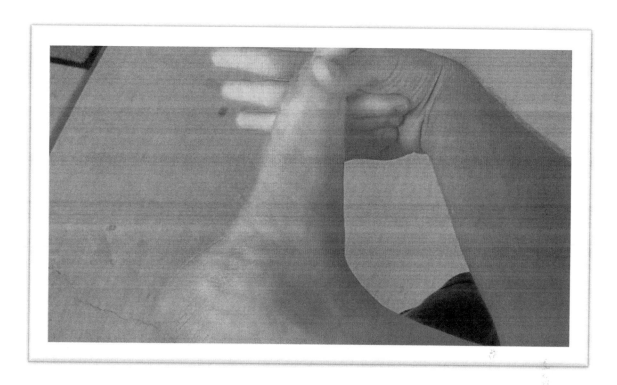

Hold for 30 seconds

Part Three

Grab all of the toes and big toe, and pull them back.

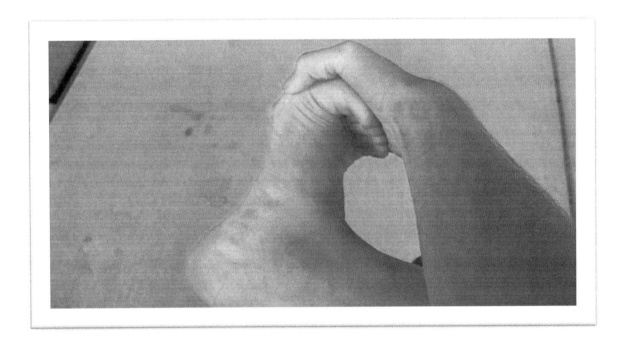

Hold for 30 seconds.

Stretch Two

This one is tough to do properly. For that reason I will show you what it looks like first. Next, read the guidelines until you understand all the steps.

<u>Stop!</u> Did you warm up yet? Be sure to get some kind of aerobic warm up before doing this section of stretches. If you are unable to bicycle or swim, walk around for a while or find some way to get your body moving and warmed up. (I understand how hard this can be when your heel hurts, but you must find a way. Obviously be sure not to hurt your heel more in the process. You can also lie on your back and imagine you're on a bicycle and pedal your feet in the air.)

Part One

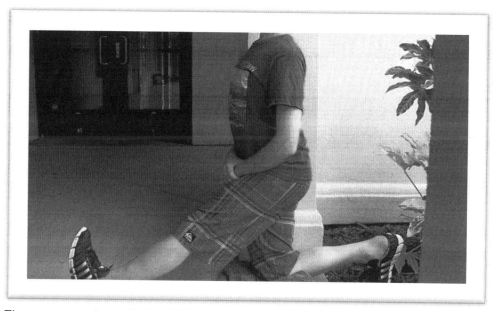

- Flex your quads really hard! This is the muscle above the knee cap. Do this by trying to make your leg as straight as possible. This causes the hamstrings to release
- Flex the shin really hard by bringing your toes to your knee
- Hips need to face forward and chest needs to be UP!
- Slowly bow forward and stick your butt out, but not too much. You shouldn't need to go that far down. Keep the chest up and work on all the steps here until you feel a stretch that goes from your toes to your back
- Do this stretch for 20 seconds, relax for 10 seconds, then hold for 30 seconds

Part Two

This one is similar, but you need to notice where the chest / hips are pointing and also where the foot points. The entire bottom of the foot will be facing towards the opposite leg being stretched.

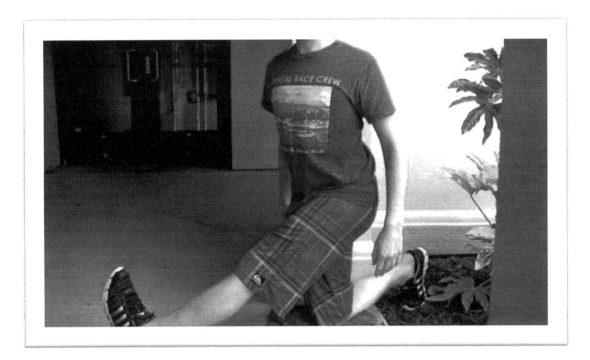

- o Flex quad muscles
- o Flex shin muscles
- o Hips need to face toward the leg being stretched
- o Foot needs to turn toward the opposite leg AND have the toes pointed towards your knee
- o Chest needs to be up and facing toward the leg being stretched
- o You will feel a long stretch on the outside part of the leg and down to the outside edge of the calf
- o Do this stretch for 20 seconds, relax for 10 seconds, then hold for 30 seconds

Part Three

This stretch is similar to the other two, but a little different. The chest needs to face away from the leg being stretched. The foot needs to be facing away from the opposite leg.

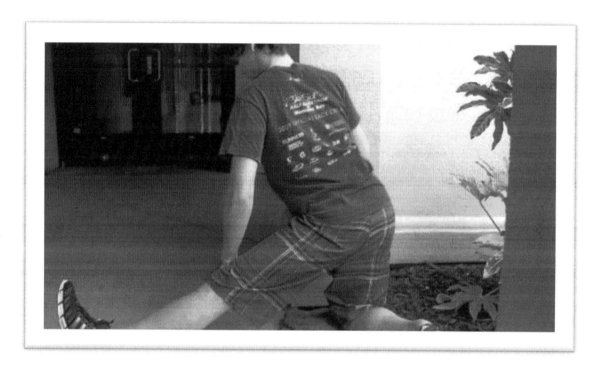

- ○ Flex quads
- ○ Flex shins
- ○ Hips Face away from the leg being stretched
- ○ Chest needs to be up
- ○ Try to push the butt out a little to deepen the stretch
- ○ Face the foot away from you. Turn it towards the outside edge of your leg
- ○ This stretch will be felt on the inside of the leg and in the hamstrings
- ○ Do this for 20 seconds, relax for 10 seconds, then do it for another 30 seconds

Stretch Three

For stretch three, we will be isolating the calf muscle. Like the last stretch, there are three parts to it. Each one needs 30 seconds of stretching. The difference in all of these stretches is where you face your foot. In the last stretch, you needed to face the foot away from your opposite leg, or towards it. For this one, same thing applies.

Part One

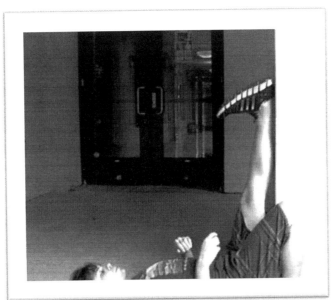

- Drive the whole leg to the ground, try to press your lower back and butt flat against the ground

- Flex the toes to the knee with some effort

- Keep the foot flat and try to pull it back with just your muscles as much as you can. For some, using a towel to pull the foot towards you can help a lot.

- The hardest part of this stretch is bringing your butt/leg down to the ground. Imagine your leg literally pushing down to the ground while still pulling your toes to your knee.

- Hold for 30 second

Part Two

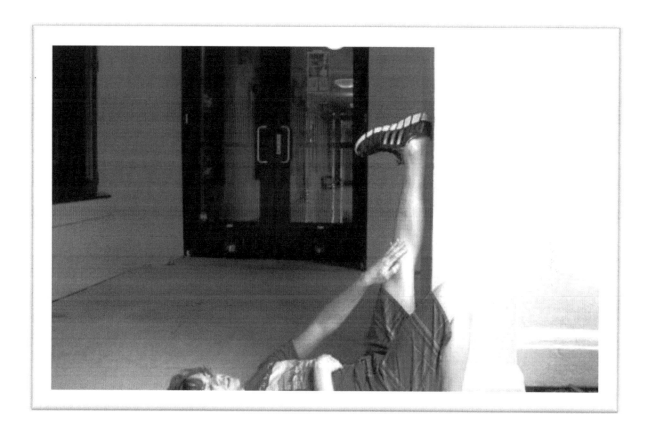

- ○ The first steps are the same as the last stretch. The main difference is that you will face the inside edge AWAY from the opposite leg.

- ○ Hold for thirty seconds

Part Three

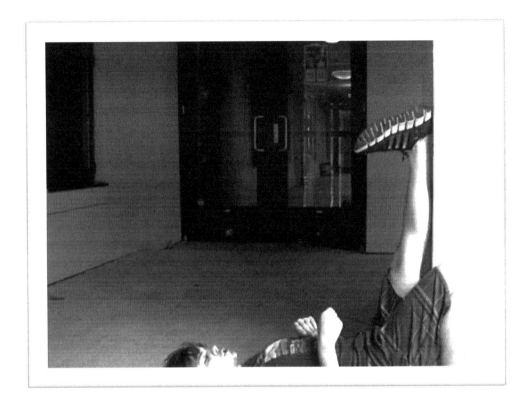

- ○ This stretch is the same as the previous two stretches, but this time you will need to face the bottom of your foot toward the opposite leg

- ○ Hold for 30 seconds

Stretch Four

This stretch is not nearly as important as the other stretches, but for some people with plantar fasciitis, this area will be causing them a lot of pain. I suggest everyone to try this stretch for a week or so and see if there is any improvement. Keep this stretch as part of your stretching routine regardless, and ease into it.

Part One

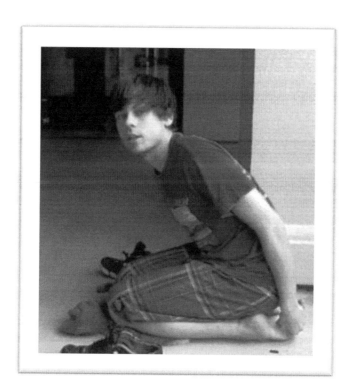

- Assume a kneeling position and then pull the big toes up toward your butt until you feel a stretch on the shin. After that, pull all the toes up as much as you can.

Part Two

This stretch is really great after you have been getting great results for a few weeks and your pain levels have improved a lot. If you have severe plantar fasciitis, this stretch can tear the heck out of your plantar fascia even more; trust me, I learned the hard way. So go easy and know that when you can do this comfortably, you are on the road to some long term recovery!

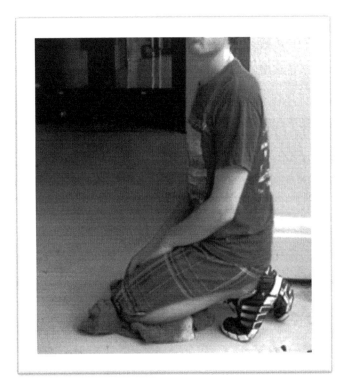

- o GO SLOW.

- o If your plantar fasciitis is severe, do not try this one until you have been doing the previous stretches for a few weeks. You can always try the stretch out, and go very gently to see how it feels. Be very careful.

- o Even if you do get rid of your plantar fasciitis, do not jump into this stretch. Do the previous stretches first EVERY time before doing this stretch.

Bonus MSTR Methods

Focused scraping massage:

This one is really neat and probably my personal favorite. It works great for really chronic plantar fasciitis and you can get some amazing results from this method alone. The tool I use is a spoon. Run the edge of the spoon back and forth RIGHT where it hurts. For me, it was a lump of scar tissue right in front of the heel. Try to find any deep lumps on the heel and rub them out with a lot of force. With this one I try to go as deep as I can. After you are done with this, you may want to ice it. You do not have to, but many people find this to be a good time to do so.

I would do this every other day if I was in a lot of pain. This technique differs from scraping in that you do not scrape the skin. You will use the edge of the spoon to dig deep into the skin and then rub the lumps without moving the spoon over the skin. The direction you want to put the spoon on the heel and the direction you want to rub are as noted on the picture on the next page.

If you feel very sore or it becomes more tender afterwards, you need to rest it for a while before trying it out again. Use common sense. If it hurts pretty bad, give it a rest. Experiment and figure out what works for you. Some may need to wait three days in between each of these sessions. Others will only need a day.

64

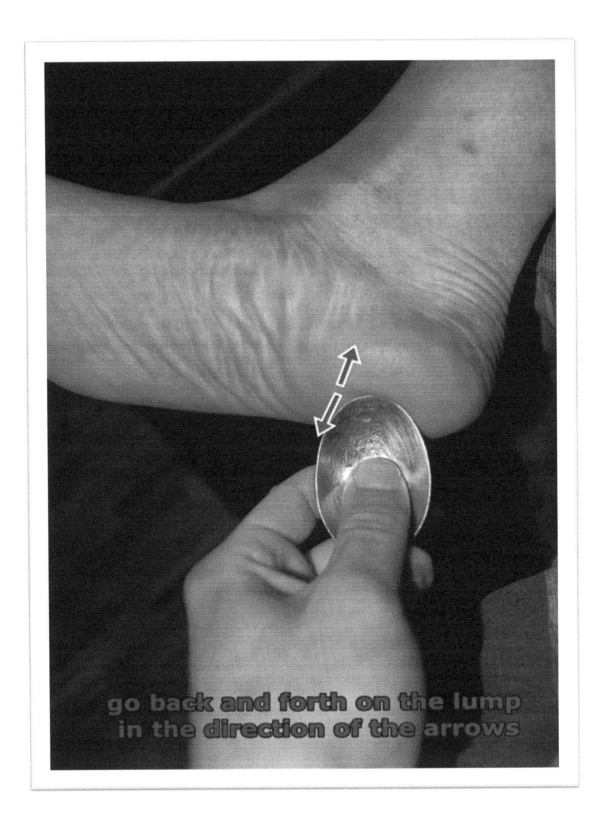

Breaking up extreme scar tissue:

The other bonus method is a modification of one of the previous methods. What you want to do is use your wooden foot roller to break up some scar tissue. Here is how I want you to approach this one:

1. Roll feet back and forth on the wooden roller SOFTLY for a few minutes. After a while, your feet will become less tender than when you started.

2. Softly roll the heel only. Feel around for any lumps. You may not feel any lumps; it may just be really tender.

3. Now I want you to press as much weight as you can into that heel. This sounds crazy to do for some of you, so don't do it too early on! But if you have been doing my methods for a while, you will start getting used to the therapies and your body will be able to take some extreme pressure on the heel. It will take a while, but you will eventually be able to press almost all of your weight on your heel.

4. ICE IT.

5. Rest for a little while, and then start moving around! After I do this one, I go back on my stationary bicycle for a while to get the blood pumping again.

Chapter 5: How to Ice

Icing can be extremely helpful when you manually break up scar tissue with massage or scraping. After a hard session, your foot can feel pretty inflamed. The best time to ice is directly after the massage. If you reinjure it badly, get ice on it as soon as possible. Use common sense though. If you feel too cold, stop icing.

Be aware that icing should not be counted on to fix your heel pain. Theoretically icing actually slows down healing (the reason inflammation makes the area warm is to speed up metabolism and boost healing speed). The reason most main stream medicine likes to use ice is because it reduces pain (by slowing down the nerve pain impulse). Understand that icing is for symptomatic relief of plantar fasciitis, but it does little to nothing when it comes to actually "fixing" the causes of plantar fasciitis.

How to ice properly:

Take an ice cube, don't cover your foot with anything, and rub the bare ice on your skin. Do this till your heel is pretty cold, but don't leave it on for more than a few minutes. Usually mine is cold after one minute or so. Don't push it. You don't want to have frost bite on top of plantar fasciitis! Most won't recommend doing this, but to me, having an ice pack with a towel around it does little to nothing. Again, if it's feeling super cold, stop!

Ice massage:

A lot of information out there says to fill a Dixie cup with water, let it freeze and then use that as an ice massage cup. What's wrong with this is someone with plantar fasciitis has to ice a few times a day, and usually is way too busy to buy Dixie cups, fill them with water, and so on. What I find to be best is to take an ice cube, and massage the edges of the ice cube into my heel. The cool thing about this is that you can buy an ice cube tray at the dollar store, much cheaper than Dixie cups every week. And when you're massaging with ice, you can push the edge of the ice into your heel for a little ice massage.

Hot and cold baths:

When I first started these, I filled two buckets with hot water and ice cold water. Then I would dunk my foot into each one for a couple minutes or until I couldn't stand it. The problem with this is not everyone has buckets around and it's hard to fill these things up and carry them when your heel is hurting. What I found to be best is to fill a bathtub with hot water, get in and relax until everything in your body warms up. This is also a great time to stretch. Then take a tray of ice cubes and set them down next to the bath tub. Stick your foot out of the water and ice your foot until it's super cold, then dunk it in the hot bath water. When you're done, you don't have to clean up much except fill the ice tray with water again.

Metal can/frozen orange juice can method:

Simply stick a can of food of some kind, or a can of orange juice in the freezer. When you use it to ice your foot, roll your foot back and forth on the can. This is a great way to ice with no mess, and the metal transfers the cold pretty well to bare skin. It is also a nice massage for the plantar fascia.

Icing brings temporary relief and can push some nutrients around, but it's not going to give you any huge amounts of relief. So now it's time to talk about taping.

Chapter 6: Taping

What kind of tape:

The kind of tape you use depends on how severe your plantar fasciitis is. If you have really bad plantar fasciitis and can't walk for more than ten minutes, you need to use either high quality white athletic tape or Leukotape. These tapes are made to not stretch, and they stand up to the daily abuse that the plantar fascia takes. Taping can be discouraging at first, and it will take you a while to learn how to tape yourself. I gave up with taping after the first few times I tried to tape. After I learned how to tape properly, I could not walk without it. Keep trying and find what works for you!

Taping guidelines:

- Use high quality athletic tape. Leukotape is the best.

- Keep trying new ways to tape and do not be discouraged if you're not finding relief. It took me a long time to teach myself how to tape my feet, but once I learned how much relief it can give me, I did it every day for eight months.

- SLOWLY peel off the tape when you're done. I have had huge chunks of skin torn off from peeling the tape off too fast. This is extremely painful, so be sure to go slowly.

- The tape isn't going to stick if the skin is not clean and dry. Use soap and water to clean it, or rubbing alcohol and a towel. Soap and water is best.

- If you have mild plantar fasciitis, you can use the stretchy types of tape such as KT tape or Spider Tech tape.

- If you have to have the tape on all day, use leukotape. It's extremely strong and I have heard of people having it on for 5 days. (I suggest taking it off at the end of the day so the skin can air out) You can also ice the foot even with it on.

- When I first started taping, I tried a cheap no name brand from a pharmacy. It didn't stick for more than a few hours and discouraged me from taping for a while. Don't do this! Buy the nice athletic tape and learn how to use that. You surely get what you pay for when it comes to athletic tape.

How to tape

This one I will only demonstrate by video. It is hard to take pictures of everything, and it is a very dynamic movement to apply the tape properly, so go online and type these into your address bar to be directed to a video tutorial

How to tape with athletic tape:
http://www.pfsurvivalguide.com/taping-for-plantar-fasciitis

How to tape with KT tape (for mild plantar fasciitis only):
http://www.pfsurvivalguide.com/kt-tape-tutorial

Chapter 7: ESWT

What ESWT does is cause a localized inflammatory response and allows the body to heal the area (hopefully to break free of the chronic inflammation). This is especially useful if you have chronic plantar fasciitis. It also encourages your body to make new blood vessels in the heel area so that more nutrients are forced into the area. If anyone says it's like ultra sound, they are only partially right. ESWT is many times more powerful and makes regular ultrasound look like a joke. I personally like ESWT, but not here in America. I traveled to Canada to get it done, and it helped a bit, but it took 4 months to see the results. It didn't seem to help my pain, but it did help how long I could stand for. Everyone's results vary when it comes to ESWT, but if you have had plantar fasciitis for at least four months, it can almost always give you positive results.

Things to keep in mind:

- Go to another country to get it done. Here in the states, I have been quoted one session being 9000 dollars! I had three sessions done in Canada for 800 dollars. I took the train and it was only 130 dollars to go there and 127 to come back. For many people, it's much cheaper to pay for a flight to Canada than it is to get the procedure done in America.

- Get the low level energy ESWT. This kind is the best. You will benefit from increased recovery time and cheaper costs.

- Do not take NSAIDs after having ESWT done. It literally makes the whole procedure worthless. ESWT's purpose is to cause more inflammation to fix what is wrong with your plantar fascia. NSAIDs stop this from happening.

- It takes from two weeks to two months for any results to show, so be patient!

- ESWT is more for chronic plantar fasciitis, so wait until you have had it for at least four months for it to be really effective.

- The procedure is very painful. The pain stops shortly after it's done, and doesn't get worse, but the initial treatment can make you scream (I did).

Chapter 8: Surgery and Cortisone Shot

Surgery:

I believe that surgeries should not be a method in treating plantar fasciitis. They have many complications and most stories I have read have been pretty bad. If you're really not seeing any results with conservative methods, I suggest finding a manual therapy / soft tissue practitioner in your area, and throw your money at them till you get out of the downward spiral.

Anti-inflammatories and the cortisone shot:

Anti-inflammatories and the cortisone shot are drugs that reduce inflammation. They have many rare side effects. I don't suggest taking any for plantar fasciitis. The reason I believe this is because if you don't feel the pain, you don't know what is hurting it more. Pain is a very important tool that tells you what to do and what not to do. The drugs only cause temporary relief. Some of the side effects of anti-inflammatories are pretty nasty as well. Medicinenet.com sums up what you need to know:

"The most serious side effects are kidney failure, liver failure, ulcers and prolonged bleeding."

More information can be found on Google. Look up whatever drug you want to use and put "side effects" after the name of the drug. I believe my liver and kidneys to be much more important than my foot, so I won't introduce those drugs into my system. With a cortisone shot, you give yourself a better chance of partially rupturing the fascia, and you could cause other complications such as causing the fat pad to atrophy.

Here's something I found at: http://orthopedics.about.com/od/footankle/a/fasciitis_2.htm:

"[…] Many physicians do not like to inject cortisone because there are potentially serious problems with cortisone injections in the heel area. The two problems that cause concern are fat pad atrophy and plantar fascial rupture. Both of these problems occur in a very small percentage of patients, but they can cause a worsening of heelpain symptoms."

Again, I don't feel that using anti-inflammatories and cortisone are worth the risk.

Chapter 10: Prolotherapy

In this chapter, I let me friend Howard Rosen M.D. tell you what you need to know about using Prolotherapy for Plantar Fasciitis:

Prolotherapy is an excellent treatment option for plantar fascitis. It involves an injection of a solution such as dextrose and local anesthesia to the affected painful area (Usually the front of the heel). The standard explanation for the effectiveness of Prolotherapy is that the Prolotherapy solution helps the body find the correct area to repair by causing a localized area of inflammation ("Good inflammation").

Prolotherapy for Plantar Fasciitis Protocol:

Ice or Cold Spray is used to help numb the heel area before any injections are performed. The smallest needle is then used to inject more local anesthesia to further anesthetize the area to be injected. After the heel is numb, Prolotherapy solutions are injected into areas that need "good inflammation".

Prolotherapy injections that are meant to reach the tip of the calcaneus (common injection area for plantar fasciitis, this is where the plantar fascia attaches to the heel bone, and is usually a problem area if you have plantar fasciitis) is started outside the heel pad, on the side of the heel. This is because it is thought that the heel pad is more susceptible to infection if injected. So instead of injecting there, we reach the plantar fascias attachment by injecting from the side of the heel.

-In summary: Anesthetize the area to be injected. When area is numb, inject Prolotherapy solutions into the problem areas that need "good inflammation". Inject the solution in from the side of the heel to avoid possibility of infection.

If the side of the heel bone is painful, this area is also injected in a similar manner. If the metatarsal bones are painful, these bones are injected too. Another Prolotherapy approach is called neural Prolotherapy. Neural Prolotherapy involves the injection of the nerves that innervate the plantar fascia.

The only solution injected is dextrose. Dextrose injected alone has been able to produce pain relief.

Another Prolotherapy treatment is the use of Prologel. Prologel is a topical cream invented by the author (Howard Rosen MD). Prologel is a patent-pending topical dextrose cream which is able to help many patients without an injection. Cheap internet ultrasound machines can be purchased for less than $30 to drive in Prologel even further. (Very cheap and safe option! No injections=No infections)

Recovery Times:

You can usually resume work the next day without complications. It depends on how many injections you have, and your underlying health disorders that may change your results. Most people are usually good to go after an injection, and walk out of the office with the same or less pain than when they walked in.

Results Time Estimate:

Prolotherapy takes time to work. If you have Neural Prolotherapy, you may have instant results. But for most, you will have to wait a bit. Some people can see results in 2 weeks. For some it can take 2 months. It is different case by case. It is good to consistently see a Prolotherapist and do what they recommend. If they think you need 2 injections, then do that and see how you feel. If they recommend 8 injections, you may very well need that many.

-Howard Rosen, M.D.

Long story short on Prolotherapy: It can give pain relief results by causing a localized "good" inflammatory reaction. This reaction causes healing and regeneration of the damage in the plantar fascia. After a few weeks or months of having this "good" inflammation, the plantar fascia is stronger with less scar tissue and more collagen.

Chapter 9: Other Therapies

Acupuncture:

I'm all for acupuncture for getting rid of the pain, but with plantar fasciitis, you need to feel the pain. You need to know what not to do so you do not injure your body more. Acupuncture also doesn't address the many other non-neurological perpetuating factors involved with plantar fasciitis. It's best to save your money and go to a trained soft tissue practitioner.

Ultrasound:

Ultrasound doesn't penetrate deep enough for it to affect the plantar fascia, so is worthless when it comes to plantar fasciitis. All it does is heat up the tissue, which increases metabolism and healing. The problem is, the plantar fascia is too deep to be touched by ultrasound, so it's worthless. Overall, I feel it's a waste of time and money.

Light therapy/LLLT (Low Level Laser Therapy):

Although I've never had this therapy done, there is good research showing why and how it works. I personally find that if you want good bang for your buck, invest in a far infrared heat lamp. Don't let the name scare you, they are easy to find and are usually around 10 dollars. It gives off light rays with the same frequency as most therapeutic lasers or therapeutic lights, and you can have this thing on you for tons of time without adverse effects. It is also a million times cheaper than seeing a specialist. I don't feel that it is a good enough therapy to "fix" plantar fasciitis, but it can help warm up the tissues before you massage or stretch them.

17898597R00045

Made in the USA
Middletown, DE
13 February 2015